The road to recovery;Post orthopedic surgery selfcare guide
Did you break a bone?Do not panic.

Keys to prevention,diagnosis,surgery,treatment and healing(rehabilitation)

Lizzy Hunt

Copyright

All rights reserved. No part of this publication may be reproduced, distributed or transmitted in any form or by any means, including photocopying, recording or other electronic or mechanical methods, without prior written permission of the publisher except in the case of brief quotations, embodied in critical reviews and certain other noncommercial uses permitted by copyright law.

Copyright © Lizzy Hunt, 2024

Disclaimer

This book is for educational purposes only and should not be used as a substitute for professional medical advice. The author and publisher make no representations or warranties about the completeness, accuracy, reliability, suitability, or applicability of the contents. The techniques, strategies, and suggestions may not be suitable for everyone, and individual results may vary. The mention of specific products or services does not imply endorsement by the author or publisher. Liability for any claims, damages, liabilities, costs, or expenses arising from the use of this book is at the reader's own risk.

Post orthopedic surgery selfcare:Lizzy Hunt

About the Author

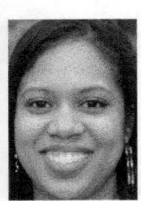

Lizzy Hunt is a healthcare professional with over a decade of experience in orthopedic care and rehabilitation. She believes in self-care and personalized rehabilitation plans, and is dedicated to sharing her knowledge. Lizzy is also a writer and educator, sharing her expertise through writing, speaking engagements, and community outreach. She has written a comprehensive guide to post-orthopedic self-care, offering practical advice, evidence-based recommendations, and an empathetic approach, making it an invaluable resource for those navigating recovery from orthopedic injuries or surgeries.

6
Post orthopedic surgery selfcare: Lizzy Hunt

Table of content

Introduction	**10**
Understanding orthopedic conditions	**13**
Common Orthopedic Injuries and Surgeries	**19**
Preparation for Recovery	**25**
Pre-operative Preparations:	25
Mental and Emotional Readiness for Surgery:	27
Immediate Post-Surgery Care	**30**
Managing Pain and Discomfort:	30
Wound Care and Infection Prevention:	31
Early Mobility Exercises:	32
Physical Rehabilitation	**35**
Importance of Physical Therapy:	35
Types of Exercises for Different Stages of Recovery:	36
Progression of Exercises and Milestones to Aim For:	37
Nutrition and Hydration in Orthopedic Recovery	**40**
Nutritional Requirements for Bone Health and Healing:	40
Foods to Promote Recovery and Reduce Inflammation:	41
Importance of Hydration in the Healing Process:	42
Pain Management in Orthopedic Recovery	**45**
Medications for Pain Relief:	45
Alternative Pain Management Techniques:	46
Assistive Devices and Adaptive Techniques in Orthopedic Recovery	**49**
Tips for Adapting Daily Activities During Recovery:	50
Mental and Emotional Well-being in Orthopedic Recovery	**54**
Coping with Limitations and Frustrations:	54
Strategies for Staying Positive and Motivated During Recovery:	55
Seeking Support from Friends, Family, or Support Groups:	56

Returning to Daily Activities in Orthopedic Recovery   59
    Gradual Reintroduction of Activities of Daily Living: 59
    Safety Precautions to Prevent Re-Injury: 60
    Resuming Work, Exercise, and Recreational Activities: 61
Long-Term Maintenance in Orthopedic Health   62
    Importance of Continued Exercise and Physical Activity: 63
    Strategies for Preventing Future Injuries: 64
Monitoring for Signs of Complications or Recurrence   66
Conclusion: 70

Introduction

Navigating Your Orthopedic Recovery Journey

Welcome to "The Road to Recovery: A Post-Orthopedic Self-Care Guide." Whether you're facing the aftermath of an injury, surgery, or chronic orthopedic condition, embarking on the path to recovery can feel like navigating uncharted territory. It's a journey that requires patience, perseverance, and a holistic approach to healing.

In these pages, you'll find a comprehensive resource designed to support you every step of the way. Drawing from my own experiences as a healthcare professional and the collective wisdom of orthopedic experts, "The Road to Recovery" is more than just a guide, it's a road map to reclaiming your mobility, restoring your strength, and revitalizing your well-being.

Orthopedic conditions can affect individuals of all ages and backgrounds, from athletes recovering from sports injuries to seniors seeking relief from joint pain. Regardless of where you find yourself on this spectrum, one thing remains constant: the importance of self-care in facilitating a successful recovery.

Throughout this book, we'll explore the essential components of post-orthopedic self-care, from practical tips for managing pain and promoting healing to strategies for maintaining your mental and emotional well-being. Each chapter is crafted to provide you with the knowledge, tools, and support you need to navigate the challenges of recovery with confidence and resilience.

But this book is more than just a manual for physical rehabilitation, it's a testament to the power of the human spirit. It's a celebration of your strength, your courage, and your unwavering determination to overcome obstacles and emerge stronger on the other side.

So, as you embark on this journey, remember that you are not alone. Whether you're taking your first tentative steps or you're well on your way to recovery, know that there is a community of support surrounding you, cheering you on every step of the way.

With dedication, perseverance, and the right tools at your disposal, there's no limit to what you can achieve. So let's embark on this journey together, and let "The Road to Recovery" be your trusted companion along the way.

Warmest regards,

Lizzy Hunt

Understanding orthopedic conditions

Orthopedic conditions encompass a wide range of musculoskeletal disorders, affecting the bones, joints, muscles, ligaments, and tendons of the body. These conditions can result from injuries, overuse, degenerative changes, or underlying medical conditions, and they often present unique challenges to those affected. By gaining a deeper understanding of orthopedic conditions, you can better comprehend their impact on the body and the principles guiding their treatment and management.

Common Orthopedic Conditions

1. **Fractures:** Fractures, or broken bones, occur when excessive force is applied to a bone, causing it to crack or break. Fractures can vary in severity, from simple fractures that require minimal intervention to complex fractures that may require surgical repair.
2. **Osteoarthritis:** Osteoarthritis is a degenerative joint disease characterized by the gradual breakdown of cartilage, the smooth tissue that cushions the ends of bones in the joints. As cartilage wears away, bones may rub against each other, leading to pain, stiffness, and loss of mobility.

3. **Tendonitis:** Tendonitis, also known as tendinitis, is inflammation or irritation of a tendon, the thick cord that attaches muscles to bones. Tendonitis commonly affects the shoulders, elbows, wrists, knees, and heels, and it can result from repetitive movements, overuse, or sudden injury.
4. **Sprains and Strains:** Sprains involve stretching or tearing of ligaments, the tough bands of tissue that connect bones to each other, while strains involve stretching or tearing of muscles or tendons. These injuries often occur during physical activity or sudden movements and can vary in severity.
5. **Cartilage Injuries:** Cartilage is the smooth, flexible tissue that cushions the ends of bones and allows for smooth movement in the joints. Injuries to cartilage, such as tears or degenerative changes, can lead to pain, swelling, and stiffness in the affected joint. Common sites for cartilage injuries include the knee (meniscal tears) and the shoulder (labral tears).

Impact on Mobility and Function

Orthopedic conditions can significantly impact an individual's mobility, function, and quality of life. Pain, stiffness, weakness, and instability are common symptoms that may limit a person's ability to perform daily activities, work, exercise, or participate in recreational pursuits.

Additionally, orthopedic conditions can affect posture, gait, and balance, increasing the risk of falls and other injuries.

Treatment Approaches

The treatment of orthopedic conditions often involves a multidisciplinary approach aimed at reducing pain, improving function, and promoting healing. Depending on the nature and severity of the condition, treatment options may include:

- **Medications:** Nonsteroidal anti-inflammatory drugs (NSAIDs), analgesics, and corticosteroids may be prescribed to alleviate pain and inflammation.
- **Physical Therapy:** Physical therapy plays a crucial role in orthopedic rehabilitation, focusing on exercises, stretches, and manual techniques to improve strength, flexibility, and mobility.
- **Orthotic Devices:** Braces, splints, orthopedic shoes, and other assistive devices may be recommended to support and stabilize affected joints or limbs.
- **Surgical Intervention:** In cases of severe trauma, instability, or degenerative changes, surgical procedures such as fracture fixation, joint replacement, or arthroscopic surgery may be necessary.

Causes of Orthopedic Injuries:

Orthopedic injuries can occur due to a variety of factors, including:

- **Trauma:** Falls, sports-related injuries, motor vehicle accidents, and other forms of trauma can cause fractures, dislocations, and soft tissue injuries.
- **Overuse:** Repetitive movements, excessive strain, and prolonged activity can lead to overuse injuries such as tendonitis, stress fractures, and muscle strains.
- **Degenerative Changes:** Aging, wear and tear, and underlying medical conditions such as osteoarthritis can contribute to degenerative changes in the musculoskeletal system, increasing the risk of injury.
- **Poor Biomechanics:** Improper body mechanics, poor posture, and biomechanical imbalances can place undue stress on the musculoskeletal system, leading to injury over time.

Prevention and Management

While some orthopedic conditions are unavoidable, there are steps you can take to reduce your risk and manage existing conditions effectively. These may include:

- Maintaining a healthy weight to reduce stress on the joints.

- Practicing proper ergonomics and body mechanics to prevent injuries during daily activities and exercise.
- Engaging in regular physical activity to strengthen muscles, improve flexibility, and support joint health.
- Using appropriate protective gear during sports and recreational activities to prevent trauma and overuse injuries.

By understanding the nature of orthopedic conditions and adopting proactive strategies for prevention and management, you can take control of your musculoskeletal health and optimize your overall well-being.

16
Post orthopedic surgery selfcare:Lizzy Hunt

Common Orthopedic Injuries and Surgeries

Orthopedic injuries encompass a broad spectrum of conditions that affect the musculoskeletal system, ranging from acute trauma to chronic degenerative changes. When conservative measures fail to provide relief or restore function, surgical intervention may be necessary to repair damaged tissues, alleviate pain, and promote healing. Below are some of the most common orthopedic injuries and surgeries:

1. Fractures and Dislocations:

- Fractures: Fractures occur when excessive force is applied to a bone, resulting in a crack or break. Common types of fractures include:
    - Closed Fracture: The bone breaks but does not penetrate the skin.
    - Open Fracture: The bone breaks through the skin, increasing the risk of infection.
    - Stress Fracture: A hairline crack in the bone caused by repetitive stress or overuse.
- Dislocations: Dislocations occur when the ends of the bones in a joint are forced out of their normal positions. Common sites for dislocations include the shoulder, elbow, hip, knee, and ankle.

2. Ligament and Tendon Injuries:

- Anterior Cruciate Ligament (ACL) Tear: A tear in the ACL, one of the major ligaments in the knee, often resulting from sudden stops, changes in direction, or direct impact.
- Rotator Cuff Tear: A tear in one or more of the muscles and tendons that stabilize the shoulder joint, commonly caused by repetitive overhead movements or trauma.
- Achilles Tendon Rupture: A partial or complete tear of the Achilles tendon, the large tendon that connects the calf muscles to the heel bone, typically occurring during activities that involve sudden acceleration or jumping.

3. Degenerative Joint Diseases:

- Osteoarthritis: Osteoarthritis is a progressive degenerative joint disease characterized by the breakdown of cartilage and the formation of bone spurs. Common sites for osteoarthritis include the knees, hips, hands, and spine.
- Rheumatoid Arthritis: Rheumatoid arthritis is an autoimmune disorder that causes chronic inflammation of the joints, leading to pain, swelling, stiffness, and joint deformity.

4. Spinal Conditions:

- Herniated Disc: A herniated disc occurs when the soft, gel-like center of a spinal disc protrudes through a tear in the outer layer, pressing on nearby nerves and causing pain, numbness, or weakness.
- Spinal Stenosis: Spinal stenosis is a narrowing of the spinal canal or neural foramina, compressing the spinal cord or nerve roots and causing symptoms such as pain, tingling, or weakness in the arms or legs.

Common Orthopedic Surgeries:

- **Fracture Fixation:** Surgical procedures to realign and stabilize fractured bones using internal fixation devices such as plates, screws, rods, or wires.
- **Arthroscopic Surgery:** Minimally invasive procedures performed with an arthroscope, a thin, flexible tube with a camera and surgical instruments, used to diagnose and treat conditions such as torn ligaments, cartilage damage, or joint inflammation.
- **Joint Replacement:** Surgical removal of damaged or diseased joint surfaces and replacement with prosthetic components made of metal, plastic, or ceramic. Common joint replacements include hip replacement, knee replacement, and shoulder replacement.

- **Ligament Reconstruction:** Surgical repair or reconstruction of torn ligaments using graft tissue or synthetic materials to restore stability and function to the affected joint.
- **Spinal Fusion:** Surgical fusion of two or more vertebrae to stabilize the spine, reduce pain, and prevent further degeneration in cases of spinal instability or deformity.

Orthopedic injuries and surgeries can have a profound impact on an individual's mobility, function, and quality of life. By understanding the nature of these conditions and the treatment options available, individuals can make informed decisions about their care and take proactive steps toward recovery and rehabilitation.

Preparation for Recovery

Preparing for recovery from an orthopedic injury or surgery is a crucial step in ensuring a smooth and successful rehabilitation process. This preparation involves not only physical considerations but also mental and emotional readiness for the challenges ahead. Let's delve into the key aspects of preparation:

Pre-operative Preparations:

Before undergoing orthopedic surgery, there are several important steps individuals can take to prepare themselves physically and mentally:

1. **Consultation with Healthcare Providers:** Schedule consultations with your orthopedic surgeon, anesthesiologist, and other members of your healthcare team to discuss the procedure, address any concerns, and ensure that you fully understand what to expect before, during, and after surgery.
2. **Medical Evaluation:** Undergo a comprehensive medical evaluation to assess your overall health and identify any pre-existing conditions that may impact your surgical outcome. This evaluation may include blood tests, imaging studies, and other diagnostic tests as recommended by your healthcare provider.

3. **Medication Management:** Review your current medications with your healthcare provider to determine which medications should be continued, discontinued, or adjusted in the days leading up to surgery. Some medications, such as blood thinners, may need to be temporarily stopped to reduce the risk of bleeding during surgery.
4. **Smoking Cessation:** If you smoke, consider quitting or reducing your smoking habits before surgery. Smoking can impair wound healing, increase the risk of complications, and prolong the recovery process. Your healthcare provider can provide resources and support to help you quit smoking.
5. **Nutrition and Hydration:** Maintain a healthy diet rich in vitamins, minerals, and protein to support your body's healing process. Stay hydrated by drinking plenty of water and avoiding excessive alcohol consumption in the days leading up to surgery.
6. **Pre-operative Exercises:** Engage in pre-operative exercises recommended by your physical therapist or healthcare provider to strengthen the muscles surrounding the affected joint and improve your range of motion. These exercises can help optimize your physical condition and facilitate post-operative recovery.
7. **Arrangements for Home Care:** Make arrangements for post-operative care and assistance at home, especially if you anticipate needing help with activities of daily living during the initial stages of recovery. This may involve enlisting the support of family members, friends, or professional caregivers.

Mental and Emotional Readiness for Surgery:

In addition to physical preparations, it's essential to address the mental and emotional aspects of undergoing orthopedic surgery:

1. **Education and Information:** Educate yourself about the surgical procedure, expected outcomes, potential risks, and post-operative rehabilitation protocols. Having a clear understanding of what to expect can alleviate anxiety and empower you to actively participate in your recovery.
2. **Emotional Support:** Seek emotional support from loved ones, friends, or support groups who can provide encouragement, reassurance, and empathy during this challenging time. Sharing your feelings and concerns with others can help alleviate stress and promote a sense of emotional well-being.
3. **Stress Management:** Practice stress-reduction techniques such as deep breathing, meditation, mindfulness, or guided imagery to calm your mind and alleviate anxiety before surgery. Engaging in activities that bring you joy and relaxation can also help distract you from pre-operative worries.
4. **Positive Mindset:** Cultivate a positive mindset and visualize a successful outcome for your surgery and recovery. Focus on the progress you can make and the improvements you can achieve with time, patience, and perseverance.

5. **Communication with Healthcare Providers:** Communicate openly and honestly with your healthcare providers about any fears, concerns, or questions you may have regarding the surgery. They can offer reassurance, address your concerns, and provide additional support as needed.

By taking proactive steps to prepare for recovery, both physically and mentally, individuals can enhance their chances of a successful outcome and a smoother rehabilitation process following orthopedic surgery. Remember that recovery is a journey, and it's essential to approach it with patience, determination, and a positive attitude.

Immediate Post-Surgery Care

The immediate period following orthopedic surgery is critical for initiating the healing process and promoting optimal recovery. During this time, focused attention on managing pain, ensuring proper wound care, and initiating early mobility exercises is essential for a successful outcome.

Managing Pain and Discomfort:

1. **Medications:** Your healthcare provider will prescribe pain medications to help manage postoperative pain. Take these medications as directed, and do not hesitate to inform your healthcare team if you experience inadequate pain relief or have concerns about medication side effects.
2. **Ice Therapy:** Applying ice packs to the surgical site can help reduce swelling and alleviate pain. Use ice packs for 20-minute intervals several times a day during the initial postoperative period, being careful to protect your skin from direct contact with the ice.
3. **Elevation:** Elevating the surgical limb above heart level can help reduce swelling and improve circulation, which can contribute to pain relief. Use pillows or cushions to support the affected limb while resting or sleeping.
4. **Compression:** Your healthcare provider may recommend wearing compression garments or wraps to minimize swelling and support

the surgical site. Follow their instructions regarding the use of compression devices to ensure optimal outcomes.
5. **Relaxation Techniques:** Practice relaxation techniques such as deep breathing, guided imagery, or progressive muscle relaxation to help alleviate muscle tension and promote overall comfort during the recovery period.

Wound Care and Infection Prevention:

1. **Follow Post-operative Instructions:** Adhere closely to the post-operative instructions provided by your healthcare provider regarding wound care, dressing changes, and activity restrictions. Follow the prescribed schedule for changing dressings and inspecting the surgical incision for signs of infection or complications.
2. **Keep the Wound Clean and Dry:** Keep the surgical incision clean and dry to prevent infection. Avoid soaking the incision in water, and refrain from applying creams, lotions, or ointments unless specifically instructed by your healthcare provider.
3. **Monitor for Signs of Infection:** Be vigilant for signs of infection, including increased redness, swelling, warmth, or drainage from the surgical site, as well as fever or chills. Contact your healthcare provider immediately if you experience any of these symptoms.

4. **Maintain Proper Nutrition and Hydration:** Eating a nutritious diet and staying hydrated can support the body's healing process and reduce the risk of infection. Ensure that you consume adequate protein, vitamins, and minerals to promote tissue repair and immune function.

Early Mobility Exercises:

1. **Range of Motion Exercises:** Begin gentle range of motion exercises for the affected joint as soon as possible after surgery, as directed by your healthcare provider or physical therapist. These exercises can help prevent stiffness and maintain flexibility in the joint.
2. **Weight-Bearing Activities:** If weight-bearing is permitted based on your surgical procedure, start with partial weight-bearing exercises and progress gradually to full weight-bearing as tolerated. Use assistive devices such as crutches, walkers, or canes as needed to support your mobility.
3. **Ambulation:** Begin walking short distances as soon as you are able, starting with assistance from a caregiver or physical therapist if necessary. Gradually increase the duration and intensity of walking exercises as you regain strength and confidence in your mobility.

4. **Physical Therapy:** Attend scheduled physical therapy sessions to receive personalized guidance and instruction on early mobility exercises, strengthening exercises, and functional activities tailored to your specific needs and goals.

By proactively managing pain and discomfort, ensuring proper wound care and infection prevention, and initiating early mobility exercises, you can lay the foundation for a successful recovery following orthopedic surgery. Be patient with yourself and follow the guidance of your healthcare team as you progress through the post-operative period, and remember that gradual improvements will contribute to long-term healing and rehabilitation.

Physical Rehabilitation

Physical rehabilitation plays a crucial role in the recovery process following orthopedic surgery or injury. Under the guidance of a physical therapist, individuals can regain strength, flexibility, and mobility, ultimately achieving optimal function and quality of life. Let's explore the key components of physical rehabilitation:

Importance of Physical Therapy:

1. **Restoration of Function:** Physical therapy aims to restore optimal function to the affected area through a combination of therapeutic exercises, manual techniques, and modalities. By addressing impairments in strength, range of motion, and mobility, physical therapy helps individuals regain independence in daily activities and improve overall quality of life.
2. **Pain Management:** Physical therapists employ various techniques to manage pain and discomfort during the rehabilitation process. Through targeted exercises, modalities such as heat, ice, or electrical stimulation, and manual therapy techniques, physical therapy can alleviate pain, reduce inflammation, and promote tissue healing.
3. **Prevention of Complications:** Physical therapy plays a crucial role in preventing complications such as muscle atrophy, joint stiffness,

and functional limitations that may arise following orthopedic surgery or injury. By addressing these issues early on, physical therapy helps minimize the risk of long-term disability and facilitates a more rapid and complete recovery.
4. **Education and Empowerment:** Physical therapists educate individuals about their condition, treatment options, and self-management strategies, empowering them to take an active role in their recovery. By providing guidance on proper body mechanics, home exercises, and activity modifications, physical therapy equips individuals with the knowledge and skills needed to optimize their outcomes and prevent future injuries.

Types of Exercises for Different Stages of Recovery:

1. **Early Stage Rehabilitation (Acute Phase):** During the early stage of recovery, the focus is on reducing pain and inflammation, promoting tissue healing, and restoring basic mobility. Exercises may include gentle range of motion exercises, isometric muscle contractions, and passive stretching to prevent stiffness and maintain joint mobility.
2. **Intermediate Stage Rehabilitation (Subacute Phase):** As healing progresses, emphasis shifts to increasing strength, endurance, and functional mobility. Exercises may include progressive resistance

training, functional activities, and proprioceptive exercises to improve balance and coordination.
3. **Advanced Stage Rehabilitation (Chronic Phase):** In the later stages of rehabilitation, the goal is to maximize strength, flexibility, and functional capacity to return to pre-injury levels of activity. Exercises may include plyometric training, agility drills, and sport-specific activities to prepare individuals for a safe return to sports, work, or recreational pursuits.

Progression of Exercises and Milestones to Aim For:

1. **Incremental Progression:** Physical therapists tailor exercise programs to each individual's unique needs, gradually progressing the intensity, duration, and complexity of exercises as tolerated. This incremental approach allows for steady gains in strength, flexibility, and function while minimizing the risk of injury or setbacks.
2. **Functional Milestones:** Throughout the rehabilitation process, individuals work toward achieving specific functional milestones that signify progress and readiness for more advanced activities. These milestones may include walking without assistive devices, climbing stairs, lifting objects of increasing weight, or performing sport-specific movements with proper technique.

3. **Patient Education:** Physical therapists educate individuals about the importance of consistency, compliance, and patience in achieving rehabilitation goals. By setting realistic expectations and celebrating small victories along the way, individuals stay motivated and engaged in their recovery journey.
4. **Long-Term Maintenance:** Even after completing formal physical therapy, individuals are encouraged to continue with home exercise programs, regular physical activity, and follow-up appointments to maintain gains achieved during rehabilitation and prevent future injuries.

By understanding the importance of physical therapy, implementing appropriate exercises for different stages of recovery, and aiming for progression and milestones, individuals can maximize their potential for recovery and regain optimal function following orthopedic surgery or injury. Collaboration with a skilled physical therapist is key to achieving successful outcomes and achieving long-term musculoskeletal health.

Nutrition and Hydration in Orthopedic Recovery

Proper nutrition and hydration play integral roles in supporting bone health, facilitating healing, and optimizing recovery following orthopedic surgery or injury. By focusing on nutrient-rich foods and adequate hydration, individuals can enhance the body's ability to repair tissues, reduce inflammation, and promote overall well-being. Let's explore the key aspects of nutrition and hydration in orthopedic recovery:

Nutritional Requirements for Bone Health and Healing:

1. Calcium and Vitamin D: Calcium is essential for bone formation and strength, while vitamin D aids in calcium absorption and utilization. Include calcium-rich foods such as dairy products, leafy greens, and fortified foods in your diet, and ensure adequate sun exposure or consider vitamin D supplementation if necessary.
2. Protein: Protein is crucial for tissue repair and muscle recovery. Include lean sources of protein such as poultry, fish, eggs, beans, and legumes in your meals to support healing and maintain muscle mass during the recovery process.
3. Omega-3 Fatty Acids: Omega-3 fatty acids have anti-inflammatory properties and may help reduce inflammation and pain associated with orthopedic injuries or conditions. Include fatty fish such as

salmon, trout, and mackerel, as well as walnuts, flaxseeds, and chia seeds in your diet to benefit from these essential fats.
4. Vitamins and Minerals: Consume a variety of fruits, vegetables, whole grains, and nuts to obtain essential vitamins and minerals such as vitamin C, vitamin K, magnesium, and zinc, which play roles in collagen synthesis, bone formation, and immune function.

Foods to Promote Recovery and Reduce Inflammation:

1. Antioxidant-Rich Foods: Antioxidants help reduce inflammation and oxidative stress in the body, promoting tissue repair and healing. Include colorful fruits and vegetables such as berries, oranges, spinach, kale, and bell peppers in your diet to benefit from their antioxidant properties.
2. Anti-inflammatory Herbs and Spices: Incorporate herbs and spices such as turmeric, ginger, garlic, and cinnamon into your meals to help reduce inflammation and alleviate pain associated with orthopedic injuries or conditions.
3. Healthy Fats: Include sources of healthy fats such as avocados, olive oil, nuts, and seeds in your diet to support cellular function, reduce inflammation, and promote overall health and well-being.
4. Hydration: Drink plenty of water throughout the day to stay hydrated and support the body's healing processes. Adequate hydration is essential for maintaining proper circulation, delivering

nutrients to injured tissues, and flushing out toxins and metabolic waste products.

Importance of Hydration in the Healing Process:

1. Tissue Healing: Hydration is essential for tissue healing and repair, as water plays a critical role in maintaining cellular integrity, facilitating nutrient transport, and supporting metabolic processes involved in wound healing.
2. Inflammation Reduction: Adequate hydration helps reduce inflammation by promoting the elimination of inflammatory byproducts and toxins from the body, thereby alleviating pain and swelling associated with orthopedic injuries or conditions.
3. Joint Lubrication: Hydration helps maintain joint lubrication and cushioning, reducing friction and wear on the cartilage and promoting joint health and mobility.
4. Overall Well-Being: Proper hydration supports overall health and well-being, helping individuals feel energized, alert, and focused during the recovery process.

In summary, prioritizing proper nutrition and hydration is essential for supporting bone health, facilitating tissue healing, and optimizing recovery following orthopedic surgery or injury. By consuming nutrient-rich foods, incorporating anti-inflammatory ingredients, and staying adequately hydrated, individuals can enhance their body's ability to repair and regenerate tissues, reduce inflammation, and promote overall well-being during the recovery process.

Pain Management in Orthopedic Recovery

Pain management is a critical aspect of orthopedic recovery, helping individuals cope with discomfort and facilitate healing following surgery or injury. While medications can provide effective relief, alternative pain management techniques such as ice therapy, heat therapy, and massage offer additional options for alleviating pain and promoting comfort. Let's explore these strategies in detail:

Medications for Pain Relief:

1. Nonsteroidal Anti-Inflammatory Drugs (NSAIDs): NSAIDs such as ibuprofen (Advil, Motrin) and naproxen (Aleve) help reduce pain and inflammation by inhibiting the production of prostaglandins, chemicals that contribute to pain and swelling. These medications are commonly used to manage mild to moderate orthopedic pain.
2. Acetaminophen: Acetaminophen (Tylenol) is a pain reliever that works by blocking pain signals in the brain. It is often used as an alternative to NSAIDs for individuals who cannot tolerate or should avoid nonsteroidal anti-inflammatory medications.
3. Opioid Analgesics: Opioid medications such as oxycodone (OxyContin), hydrocodone (Vicodin), and morphine may be prescribed for severe pain following orthopedic surgery or trauma.

These medications should be used cautiously due to the risk of dependence, tolerance, and adverse effects.
4. **Muscle Relaxants:** Muscle relaxants such as cyclobenzaprine (Flexeril) or baclofen (Lioresal) may be prescribed to relieve muscle spasms and tension associated with orthopedic injuries or conditions.
5. **Topical Analgesics:** Topical analgesic creams, gels, or patches containing ingredients such as lidocaine, menthol, or capsaicin can provide localized pain relief when applied directly to the affected area.

Alternative Pain Management Techniques:

1. **Ice Therapy (Cryotherapy):** Applying ice packs or cold therapy devices to the affected area helps reduce pain, inflammation, and swelling by constricting blood vessels and numbing nerve endings. Ice therapy is particularly effective during the acute phase of injury or immediately following orthopedic surgery.
2. **Heat Therapy (Thermotherapy):** Heat therapy, such as warm compresses, heating pads, or warm baths, helps relax muscles, increase blood flow, and alleviate stiffness and discomfort

associated with orthopedic conditions. Heat therapy is beneficial for chronic pain or muscle tension.
3. Massage Therapy: Massage therapy involves kneading, stroking, or applying pressure to soft tissues to promote relaxation, reduce muscle tension, and relieve pain. Massage can improve circulation, enhance tissue flexibility, and stimulate the release of endorphins, natural pain-relieving chemicals in the body.
4. Acupuncture: Acupuncture is a traditional Chinese therapy that involves inserting thin needles into specific points on the body to stimulate nerve pathways and promote pain relief. Acupuncture may be beneficial for reducing pain and improving mobility in individuals with orthopedic conditions such as osteoarthritis or chronic back pain.
5. Transcutaneous Electrical Nerve Stimulation (TENS): TENS therapy involves applying low-voltage electrical currents to the skin via electrode pads, which helps disrupt pain signals traveling to the brain and promotes the release of endorphins. TENS therapy can provide temporary pain relief for individuals with orthopedic pain.

By combining medications for pain relief with alternative pain management techniques such as ice therapy, heat therapy, massage, and other complementary therapies, individuals can effectively manage orthopedic pain, promote comfort, and enhance their overall well-being during the recovery process. It's essential to work closely with healthcare providers to develop a comprehensive pain management plan tailored to individual needs and preferences.

Assistive Devices and Adaptive Techniques in Orthopedic Recovery

Introduction to mobility aids such as crutches, walkers, or canes, as well as tips for adapting daily activities during recovery, are essential components of orthopedic rehabilitation. These tools and techniques help individuals regain independence, mobility, and confidence as they navigate the challenges of recovery. Let's explore them in detail:

Introduction to Mobility Aids:

1. Crutches: Crutches are commonly used to provide support and stability when walking or bearing weight on an injured or recovering lower extremity. There are various types of crutches, including axillary crutches, forearm crutches, and platform crutches, each offering different levels of support and comfort. Proper fitting and training in crutch use are essential to ensure safety and effectiveness.
2. Walkers: Walkers are sturdy, four-legged devices designed to provide support and stability for individuals with balance impairments or lower extremity weakness. There are different types of walkers, including standard walkers with or without wheels,

rolling walkers (rollators), and knee walkers (scooters). Walkers offer stability and support while walking and can be customized with accessories such as baskets or trays for added convenience.
3. Canes: Canes are single-pointed devices used to provide balance and support while walking, particularly for individuals with mild to moderate mobility limitations. Canes come in various styles, including straight canes, offset canes, and quad canes, each offering different levels of stability and weight-bearing assistance. Proper sizing and positioning of the cane are crucial for optimal support and comfort.

Tips for Adapting Daily Activities During Recovery:

1. Modify Your Environment: Make modifications to your home environment to accommodate your mobility aids and ensure safety and accessibility during recovery. Remove obstacles, secure rugs and carpets, install grab bars or handrails in key areas, and arrange furniture to create clear pathways for movement.
2. Use Assistive Devices Appropriately: Familiarize yourself with the proper use of your mobility aid, whether it's crutches, a walker, or a

cane. Practice using the device under the guidance of a healthcare professional to ensure proper technique and minimize the risk of falls or injuries.
3. Pace Yourself: Take breaks as needed and avoid overexertion during daily activities. Listen to your body and prioritize rest and relaxation to conserve energy and promote healing. Use your mobility aid for support when standing or walking for extended periods.
4. Adapt Activities of Daily Living: Modify daily activities to reduce strain on your recovering joints or muscles. Use adaptive equipment such as long-handled reachers, shower stools, or dressing aids to perform tasks more easily and independently. Break tasks into smaller, manageable steps and enlist assistance from family members or caregivers as needed.
5. Practice Good Body Mechanics: Maintain proper posture and body mechanics to prevent strain or injury during daily activities. Use your legs to lift heavy objects, avoid twisting or bending at the waist, and distribute weight evenly when carrying loads to minimize stress on your joints and muscles.
6. Stay Active Within Limits: Stay active within the limits of your mobility and comfort level, engaging in gentle exercises and activities recommended by your healthcare provider or physical therapist. Focus on low-impact activities such as swimming,

cycling, or gentle stretching to maintain mobility, strength, and cardiovascular fitness during recovery.

By introducing mobility aids such as crutches, walkers, or canes and adopting adaptive techniques for daily activities, individuals can navigate the challenges of orthopedic recovery with greater confidence and independence. It's essential to work closely with healthcare professionals to determine the most appropriate assistive devices and strategies for your specific needs and goals. With patience, persistence, and proper support, you can successfully adapt to life during recovery and achieve optimal outcomes.

Mental and Emotional Well-being in Orthopedic Recovery

Maintaining mental and emotional well-being during orthopedic recovery is as crucial as physical rehabilitation. Coping with limitations and frustrations, staying positive and motivated, and seeking support from friends, family, or support groups are essential strategies for navigating the emotional challenges of recovery. Let's explore these aspects in detail:

Coping with Limitations and Frustrations:

1. Acknowledge Your Feelings: It's normal to experience a range of emotions, including frustration, sadness, or anxiety, when faced with limitations due to injury or surgery. Acknowledge your feelings and allow yourself to express them in a healthy way, whether through journaling, talking to a trusted friend or therapist, or engaging in creative outlets.
2. Focus on What You Can Control: While there may be aspects of your recovery that are beyond your control, focus on the things you can control, such as following your treatment plan, practicing self-care, and maintaining a positive mindset. Channel your energy

into activities that promote healing and well-being, rather than dwelling on limitations or setbacks.
3. Set Realistic Expectations: Be realistic about your recovery timeline and the progress you can expect to make. Understand that healing takes time and that there may be ups and downs along the way. Set achievable goals for yourself and celebrate small victories as you progress toward recovery.

Strategies for Staying Positive and Motivated During Recovery:

1. Cultivate a Positive Mindset: Focus on the silver linings and opportunities for growth that may arise from your recovery journey. Practice gratitude for the support and resources available to you, and remind yourself of your resilience and ability to overcome challenges.
2. Visualize Success: Use visualization techniques to imagine yourself achieving your goals and returning to activities you enjoy. Visualizing positive outcomes can boost confidence, motivation, and resilience during challenging times.

3. Stay Engaged and Connected: Stay connected with friends, family, and activities that bring you joy and fulfillment. Engage in hobbies, interests, and social interactions that uplift your spirits and provide a sense of normalcy and connection during recovery.
4. Focus on Self-Care: Prioritize self-care activities that nurture your physical, emotional, and mental well-being. Practice relaxation techniques such as deep breathing, meditation, or mindfulness to reduce stress and promote relaxation.

Seeking Support from Friends, Family, or Support Groups:

1. Communicate Your Needs: Don't hesitate to communicate your needs and concerns with your loved ones, friends, or healthcare providers. Let them know how they can best support you during your recovery, whether it's providing assistance with daily tasks, offering emotional support, or simply being there to listen.
2. Lean on Your Support Network: Lean on your support network for encouragement, companionship, and practical assistance during your recovery journey. Allow yourself to accept help and support from others, recognizing that it's okay to rely on others during challenging times.
3. Join a Support Group: Consider joining a support group for individuals going through similar experiences with orthopedic injuries or surgeries. Support groups provide a safe space to share

experiences, exchange advice, and offer mutual encouragement and understanding.
4. Stay Connected Virtually: If in-person support is limited, stay connected with friends, family, or support groups virtually through phone calls, video chats, or online forums. Virtual connections can provide valuable support and companionship, even when physical distancing is necessary.

By coping with limitations and frustrations, employing strategies for staying positive and motivated, and seeking support from friends, family, or support groups, individuals can navigate the emotional challenges of orthopedic recovery with resilience and strength. Remember that recovery is a journey, and it's okay to ask for help and support along the way. With patience, perseverance, and support, you can overcome obstacles and emerge stronger on the other side of your recovery journey.

Returning to Daily Activities in Orthopedic Recovery

Returning to daily activities following orthopedic surgery or injury requires a gradual reintroduction of tasks, adherence to safety precautions, and careful consideration of when and how to resume work, exercise, and recreational activities. Let's explore these aspects in detail:

Gradual Reintroduction of Activities of Daily Living:

1. Start Slowly: Begin by gradually reintroducing basic activities of daily living, such as self-care tasks (bathing, dressing), household chores (cooking, cleaning), and mobility activities (walking, climbing stairs). Pace yourself and listen to your body's signals to avoid overexertion.
2. Use Adaptive Equipment: Utilize assistive devices or adaptive equipment as needed to support your recovery and make daily tasks more manageable. This may include using grab bars in the bathroom, adaptive utensils for eating, or ergonomic tools for household chores.
3. Modify Activities: Modify activities to reduce strain on the recovering area and minimize the risk of re-injury. Break tasks into smaller, manageable steps, alternate between sitting and standing

positions, and use proper body mechanics to prevent undue stress on your joints and muscles.

Safety Precautions to Prevent Re-Injury:

1. Follow Post-operative Guidelines: Adhere closely to the post-operative instructions provided by your healthcare provider, including restrictions on weight-bearing, range of motion, and activity level. Avoid activities that may exacerbate pain or compromise healing, and seek guidance if you have any questions or concerns.
2. Use Proper Body Mechanics: Practice proper body mechanics and lifting techniques to prevent strain or injury during daily activities. Bend at the knees, keep your back straight, and lift with your legs rather than your back when lifting objects or performing tasks that require physical exertion.
3. Avoid High-Risk Activities: Steer clear of high-impact or high-risk activities that may increase the likelihood of re-injury, such as heavy lifting, contact sports, or activities that require sudden movements or twisting motions. Choose low-impact, joint-friendly activities that support your recovery goals and minimize stress on your musculoskeletal system.

Resuming Work, Exercise, and Recreational Activities:

1. Return to Work: Consult with your healthcare provider and employer to determine when it's safe and appropriate to return to work following orthopedic surgery or injury. Consider factors such as the physical demands of your job, the availability of accommodations or modifications, and your overall recovery progress.
2. Gradual Exercise Progression: Gradually reintroduce exercise and physical activity into your routine, starting with low-impact, gentle activities and gradually increasing intensity, duration, and frequency as tolerated. Focus on exercises that target the affected area while also addressing overall strength, flexibility, and cardiovascular fitness.
3. Listen to Your Body: Pay attention to your body's signals and adjust your activity level accordingly. If you experience pain, discomfort, or fatigue during or after activities, scale back or modify your routine to avoid overexertion and prevent re-injury.
4. Consult with Professionals: Consider working with a physical therapist, personal trainer, or rehabilitation specialist to develop a personalized exercise program tailored to your specific needs, goals, and recovery timeline. These professionals can provide guidance, support, and feedback to help you progress safely and effectively.

Returning to daily activities following orthopedic surgery or injury requires patience, persistence, and a gradual approach. By following post-operative guidelines, adhering to safety precautions, and gradually reintroducing work, exercise, and recreational activities, individuals can promote healing, minimize the risk of re-injury, and achieve a successful recovery outcome. Always consult with your healthcare provider before making any significant changes to your activity level or routine, and prioritize self-care and injury prevention throughout the recovery process.

Long-Term Maintenance in Orthopedic Health

Long-term maintenance is essential for sustaining orthopedic health and preventing future injuries. This involves the ongoing commitment to regular exercise and physical activity, as well as the implementation of strategies to mitigate the risk of recurrent injuries. Let's delve into these aspects:

Importance of Continued Exercise and Physical Activity:

1. Maintaining Strength and Flexibility: Regular exercise and physical activity help maintain muscle strength, joint flexibility, and overall mobility, reducing the risk of musculoskeletal imbalances and dysfunction that can contribute to injury.

2. Supporting Joint Health: Weight-bearing activities such as walking, jogging, or resistance training promote bone density and joint stability, reducing the risk of conditions like osteoporosis and osteoarthritis. Low-impact exercises such as swimming or cycling are also beneficial for joint health without placing undue stress on the joints.
3. Improving Balance and Coordination: Balance and coordination exercises, such as yoga, tai chi, or Pilates, help improve proprioception and body awareness, reducing the risk of falls and injuries, especially in older adults.
4. Managing Weight: Regular physical activity contributes to weight management by burning calories and maintaining metabolic health. Maintaining a healthy weight reduces the strain on joints and lowers the risk of obesity-related orthopedic conditions such as joint pain and arthritis.

Strategies for Preventing Future Injuries:

1. Proper Warm-Up and Cool-Down: Always begin your exercise sessions with a proper warm-up to prepare your muscles and joints for activity and reduce the risk of injury. Similarly, include a

cool-down period to gradually lower your heart rate and stretch your muscles to prevent stiffness and soreness.
2. Cross-Training: Incorporate a variety of exercises and activities into your routine to prevent overuse injuries and promote overall fitness. Cross-training allows you to work different muscle groups and engage in different movement patterns, reducing the risk of repetitive strain injuries.
3. Focus on Technique: Pay attention to proper form and technique during exercise and activities to avoid unnecessary stress on your joints and muscles. If you're unsure about the correct technique, consider working with a certified personal trainer or fitness professional for guidance.
4. Listen to Your Body: Be attentive to signs of fatigue, pain, or discomfort during exercise, and modify or stop activities as needed to prevent injury. Pushing through pain or ignoring warning signs can lead to overuse injuries and exacerbate existing conditions.
5. Gradual Progression: Progress your exercise intensity, duration, and frequency gradually over time to allow your body to adapt and reduce the risk of overuse injuries. Avoid sudden increases in intensity or volume that can overwhelm your body's capacity for recovery.
6. Maintain Good Posture: Practice good posture during daily activities and exercises to reduce strain on your spine and joints. Avoid prolonged sitting or standing in awkward positions and

incorporate exercises that strengthen postural muscles, such as core and back exercises.

By prioritizing continued exercise and physical activity and implementing strategies for preventing future injuries, individuals can promote long-term orthopedic health and well-being. Remember to consult with healthcare professionals or fitness experts for personalized recommendations and guidance tailored to your specific needs and goals. With a proactive approach to orthopedic maintenance, you can enjoy a lifetime of movement, strength, and vitality.

Monitoring for Signs of Complications or Recurrence

Vigilant monitoring for signs of complications or recurrence is crucial for individuals recovering from orthopedic injuries or surgeries. Early detection of potential issues allows for prompt intervention and treatment, minimizing the impact on recovery and preventing further complications. Here's how to effectively monitor for signs of complications or recurrence:

1. Follow-Up Appointments:

- Attend all scheduled follow-up appointments with your healthcare provider to assess your progress and monitor for any signs of complications or recurrence.
- Your healthcare provider will conduct physical examinations, review imaging studies (such as X-rays or MRIs), and discuss any changes in symptoms or functional status since your last visit.

2. Watch for Warning Signs:

- Be vigilant for any new or worsening symptoms that may indicate a complication or recurrence of your orthopedic condition.

- Common warning signs include increased pain, swelling, redness, warmth, or drainage from the surgical site, as well as loss of function, decreased range of motion, or instability in the affected joint.

3. Monitor Activity Levels:

- Pay attention to how your body responds to activity and exercise. If you experience excessive pain, fatigue, or discomfort during or after physical exertion, it may indicate a problem that warrants further evaluation.
- Gradually increase activity levels as tolerated, but avoid pushing through pain or overexerting yourself, as this can increase the risk of complications or recurrence.

4. Assess Healing Progress:

- Monitor the progress of your healing process, paying attention to the gradual resolution of symptoms and improvement in function over time.
- If you notice any delays or setbacks in your recovery, such as stalled progress or worsening symptoms, inform your healthcare provider promptly for further assessment.

5. Communicate with Your Healthcare Team:

- Maintain open and transparent communication with your healthcare team regarding any concerns, questions, or changes in your condition.
- Report any new or unusual symptoms, changes in pain intensity or quality, or other issues that arise between follow-up appointments.

6. Adhere to Rehabilitation Protocols:

- Follow the prescribed rehabilitation protocols and activity restrictions provided by your healthcare provider or physical therapist.
- Adherence to rehabilitation guidelines helps optimize healing, prevent complications, and reduce the risk of recurrence by promoting gradual, structured progression of activities.

7. Seek Prompt Medical Attention:

- If you experience any concerning symptoms or signs of complications, do not hesitate to seek prompt medical attention.
- Early intervention is key to preventing complications from worsening and improving the likelihood of successful treatment outcomes.

By actively monitoring for signs of complications or recurrence, individuals can play an active role in their recovery and collaborate with their healthcare team to address any issues that arise promptly. Remember that early detection and intervention are critical for optimizing outcomes and minimizing the impact of potential complications on your orthopedic health.

Conclusion:

As we reach the end of this comprehensive guide to post-orthopedic self-care, it's essential to reflect on the key points covered and provide encouragement for your ongoing recovery journey.

Throughout this book, we've explored a range of topics designed to support you in your recovery from orthopedic injuries or surgeries. From understanding orthopedic conditions and preparing for surgery to navigating post-operative care, rehabilitation, and long-term maintenance, each chapter has offered valuable insights, practical tips, and strategies for promoting healing, preventing complications, and optimizing your orthopedic health.

Recapping key points from the book, we've emphasized the importance of:

- Following post-operative guidelines and rehabilitation protocols provided by your healthcare team.
- Incorporating regular exercise and physical activity to promote strength, flexibility, and joint health.

- Practicing self-care techniques such as proper nutrition, hydration, and pain management to support your recovery process.
- Monitoring for signs of complications or recurrence and seeking prompt medical attention when needed.
- Gradually reintroducing daily activities and work, exercise, and recreational pursuits in a safe and structured manner.

As you continue on your recovery journey, remember that healing is a gradual process that requires patience, persistence, and dedication. Embrace each step of the journey, celebrate your progress, and stay focused on your goals. Surround yourself with a supportive network of family, friends, and healthcare professionals who can provide encouragement, guidance, and assistance along the way.

Above all, maintain a positive mindset and believe in your ability to overcome challenges and achieve optimal outcomes. Your resilience, determination, and commitment to your orthopedic health will serve as powerful catalysts for success.

As you close this book and embark on the next phase of your recovery journey, know that you are not alone. You have the knowledge, resources, and support you need to navigate the challenges ahead and emerge stronger, healthier, and more empowered than ever before.

Wishing you continued progress, resilience, and well-being on your path to recovery. You've got this!

www.ingramcontent.com/pod-product-compliance
Lightning Source LLC
Chambersburg PA
CBHW070415230526
45471CB00006B/2815